Daily Affirmations
for
Cancer Patients

Unlock the power of your subconscious mind
in your healing journey.

Ecstatic Press

Table of Contents

This book is dedicated to all those brave souls battling cancer. We recognize the challenges, uncertainties, and emotional toll of a cancer diagnosis. Through the daily 5-minute morning and evening sessions of positive affirmations, we hope to provide a tool to support your healing journey. We dedicate this book to you with admiration for your courage, strength, and perseverance, and offer it to serve as a source of inspiration, motivation, and positivity in your healing journey.

Introduction

A cancer diagnosis can turn your life upside down, but it doesn't have to take away your hope, spirit, and resilience. Belief and positive thinking are essential components of the healing journey, and positive affirmations are a powerful tool that can help us cultivate the right mindset and attitude to overcome cancer. That's why we created a book that offers fourteen 5-minute evening and morning sessions designed to last a full week. You can continue reading and repeating the affirmations each week for as long as needed to assist you in your battle to heal from cancer.

Positive affirmations are short, powerful statements that affirm your beliefs, values, and goals. When you repeat them, you tap into the power of your subconscious mind and send a clear message to your body that you are ready to heal. Belief and positive thinking are essential components of our healing journey. When we believe in our body's ability to heal and focus on positive thoughts, we activate our body's natural healing response. The placebo effect is a prime example of the power of belief and positive thinking. When we believe that a treatment will work, it often does, even if the treatment itself is not active.

The mind-body connection is a well-established phenomenon in modern medicine, and many healthcare practitioners recognize the importance of incorporating positive affirmations into cancer treatment. Studies have shown that cancer patients who practice positive affirmations experience less anxiety, depression, and pain, and have a more positive outlook on life.

This book of positive affirmations is a powerful tool that can help you cultivate the right mindset and attitude to overcome cancer. Each affirmation emphasizes a specific theme, such as faith, trust, gratitude, healing, and self-love. When you read these affirmations, focus on the words and feel the positive emotions associated with them. Visualize yourself as healthy, vibrant, and free of cancer.

It is important to remember that positive affirmations alone are not a substitute for medical treatment. Positive affirmations should be used in conjunction with a comprehensive cancer treatment plan prescribed by your healthcare provider. Positive affirmations are a complementary tool that can help support your healing journey and enhance the effectiveness of your medical treatment.

As you read this book, remember that you are not alone. There are millions of people who have overcome cancer and are living healthy, fulfilling lives. You too can be one of them. You have the power to believe in your body's ability to heal, focus on positive thoughts, and take control of your healing journey.

Cancer is a life-changing experience, but it doesn't have to be a life-ending one. The power of belief and positive thinking can help you overcome the challenges of cancer and lead a fulfilling, healthy life. This book of positive affirmations is a powerful tool that can help you cultivate the right mindset and attitude to overcome cancer. Remember, you have the power to believe in your body's ability to heal. With this book, you can make positive affirmations a part of your daily routine, and let the power of positivity assist you on your journey to healing.

Benefits Of Positive Affirmations

Positive affirmations are a powerful tool that can help cancer patients in their healing process in numerous ways, including:

- **Reduced stress and anxiety:** Positive affirmations can help reduce stress and anxiety, which are common among cancer patients. Stress can suppress the immune system, while positive affirmations can help stimulate the body's natural healing response.

- **Improved mental health:** Cancer patients often experience depression, fear, and uncertainty. Positive affirmations can help improve mental health by promoting positive emotions and reducing negative ones.

- **Increased sense of control:** A cancer diagnosis can leave patients feeling powerless and out of control. Positive affirmations can help cancer patients regain a sense of control over their lives and their healing journey.

- **Enhanced optimism:** Positive affirmations can help promote a more optimistic outlook on life, which can help cancer patients feel more hopeful and optimistic about their future.

- **Improved self-esteem:** Cancer can take a toll on a patient's self-esteem, but positive affirmations can help boost confidence and self-worth.

- **Better sleep:** Positive affirmations can help promote better sleep, which is essential for healing and recovery.

- **Increased motivation:** Positive affirmations can help increase motivation and encourage cancer patients to take an active role in their healing journey.

- **Enhanced coping skills:** Cancer patients often face numerous challenges, including physical, emotional, and financial challenges. Positive affirmations can help cancer patients develop better coping skills and increase resilience.

- **Improved quality of life:** Positive affirmations can help cancer patients experience a better quality of life by reducing stress, promoting positive emotions, and enhancing overall well-being.

In summary, positive affirmations can play a crucial role in the healing process for cancer patients. They can help reduce stress and anxicty, improve mental health, increase sense of control, enhance optimism, boost self-esteem, improve sleep, increase motivation, enhance coping skills, and improve overall quality of life.

10 Steps for Best Results

Here are 10 steps to achieve the best results in using this book to help in the healing process:

1. Five minutes in the morning and evening: To make the practice of affirmations even more accessible and effective, this book has been thoughtfully divided into 14 sessions, each lasting approximately 5 minutes. We recommend that you spend just 5 minutes each morning and another 5 minutes before going to sleep, reading and repeating these affirmations. This way, you'll start your day on a positive note, priming your mind for success and end your day with reflection and gratitude, reinforcing the positive changes you are cultivating.

2. Find a quiet and comfortable place: To get the most out of the positive affirmations in the book, find a quiet and comfortable place where you can read without distractions.

3. Choose a specific time: Choose a specific time for your morning and evening sessions, and make it a regular part of your daily routine. Consistency is key to achieving the best results.

4. Read actively: Read the positive affirmations actively and focus on the words and the emotions they evoke. Try to visualize yourself as already having achieved the desired outcome.

5. Repeat affirmations: Repeat the affirmations in your mind as you read the book. This will help reinforce the positive messages and enhance the effectiveness of the affirmations.

6. Believe: Believe that the positive affirmations are true and have faith that they will come true. Let go of any doubts or negative thoughts, and focus on positive outcomes.

7. Stay present: Stay present in the moment and focus on the positive emotions that the affirmations evoke. Avoid getting distracted by negative thoughts or worries about the future.

8. Make it a habit: Consistency is key to achieving the best results. Make reading the book of daily 5-minute morning and evening sessions of positive affirmations a habit and a regular part of your daily routine.

9. Use affirmations as a complement to medical treatment: Positive affirmations should be used as a complementary tool to medical treatment prescribed by your healthcare provider. Positive affirmations are not a substitute for medical treatment but can help enhance the effectiveness of your treatment.

Using this book of Daily 5-minute morning and evening sessions of positive affirmations can be a powerful tool to help in the healing process. To achieve the best results, find a quiet and comfortable place, choose a specific time, read actively, repeat affirmations, believe, stay present, practice gratitude, make it a habit, and use affirmations as a complement to medical treatment. By incorporating these steps into your daily practice, you can tap into the power of positive affirmations to help support your healing journey.

Let's begin.

Day 1 - Morning Affirmations

Say the following affirmations out loud, two or three times with increasing conviction and belief.

- I have the power to overcome any obstacle.
- I am filled with love, peace, and positivity every day.
- I am strong enough to fight this battle.
- I am worthy of love and support during this time.
- My body is resilient and capable of healing.
- A higher power is guiding me towards health and wellness.
- My body is a miracle, and I am grateful for it every day.
- Every cell in my body is becoming stronger and healthier.
- I am capable of finding meaning and purpose in life.
- A higher power is helping me to stay positive and optimistic.
- My body is healing, and I am becoming more energized every day.
- Every cell in my body is working to restore health and vitality.
- I am strong, resilient, and capable of overcoming anything.
- A higher power is filling me with hope and faith.
- I am surrounded by people who care for me.
- I am grateful for each day I am alive.
- I am healing and transforming into a healthier, happier person.
- My body is a temple of health and vitality.
- I am grateful for the beauty and wonder of the world.
- I am filled with gratitude for the moments of connection with others.
- I am healing and releasing stress and tension.
- My body is healing and becoming stronger with each passing day.
- I am grateful for the moments of peace and serenity.
- I am strong, resilient, and capable of overcoming adversity.
- I am grateful for the love and support of my friends.
- I am filled with gratitude for the moments of laughter and joy.
- I am healing and nourishing my body with healthy foods and thoughts.
- My body is strong, healthy, and full of energy.
- I am grateful for the love and kindness of strangers.
- I am strong, brave, and confident in my ability to heal.

Day 1 - Evening Affirmations

Say the following affirmations out loud, two or three times with increasing conviction and belief.

- I am healing and embracing a mindset of gratitude and positivity.
- My body is healing and becoming stronger with each passing moment.
- I am more than my diagnosis.
- I am brave and courageous in the face of adversity.
- I am taking one day at a time.
- My spirit is unbreakable.
- I am hopeful for a bright future.
- My body is working hard to heal itself.
- I am grateful for the little things in life.
- I am surrounded by positivity and hope.
- I am surrounded by people who lift me up.
- Every cell in my body is becoming healthier and stronger.
- I am filled with love, gratitude, and joy every day.
- My DNA is responding to the power of positive affirmations.
- Miracles happen when I stay focused on my goals.
- Every cell in my body is filled with the power to heal.
- I am capable of finding peace and serenity in any circumstance.
- My DNA is working to restore health and vitality to my body.
- Miracles happen when I believe in myself and my ability to heal.
- Every cell in my body is filled with the power of love and positivity.
- I am strong, brave, and confident in my ability to heal.
- I am filled with strength and determination.
- I am grateful for the love and support of my family.
- I am resilient and can handle anything that comes my way.
- I am surrounded by light and positivity.
- I am filled with gratitude for each day.
- My journey is unique and special.
- I am surrounded by hope and positivity.
- I am healing and taking care of my mind, body, and soul.
- My body is fighting and winning this battle.

Day 2 - Morning Affirmations

Say the following affirmations out loud, two or three times with increasing conviction and belief.

- I am grateful for the beauty and goodness in life.
- I am strong, brave, and unstoppable in the face of adversity.
- I am healing and recovering with each passing moment.
- My body is a miraculous creation, capable of incredible things.
- I am grateful for the moments of joy and happiness.
- I am filled with gratitude for the blessings in my life.
- I am grateful for the support of my friends.
- My body is healing every day.
- I am surrounded by love and encouragement.
- I am worthy of happiness and joy.
- I am surrounded by hope and optimism.
- I am surrounded by people who inspire me.
- I am grateful for the support of my community.
- I am filled with courage and strength.
- My body is capable of healing itself.
- I am grateful for the small victories.
- I am surrounded by positivity and light.
- I am filled with hope for a brighter future.
- I am surrounded by love and positivity.
- I am grateful for the moments of peace and calm.
- I can feel the power of positive relationships and connections.
- The universe is bringing me the right people and resources to help me heal.
- Every day, I am filled with the hope and optimism of a brighter future.
- I am capable of finding strength and courage within myself.
- I can feel the healing power of music, art, and nature around me.
- The universe is supporting me in my journey towards health and wellness.
- I am strong, brave, and capable of transforming my life.
- I have faith in my body's ability to heal.
- My higher power is guiding me towards health and wellness.
- I am surrounded by people who believe in me.

Day 2 - Evening Affirmations

Say the following affirmations out loud, two or three times with increasing conviction and belief.

- I trust that I am on the right path towards peace and wellness.
- I am surrounded by the beauty and wonder of the world.
- I have faith in the power of meditation and mindfulness.
- My higher power is filling me with hope and optimism.
- I am strong, resilient, and capable of transforming my life.
- I have faith in the power of creativity and expression.
- I am filled with gratitude for my loved ones.
- I am surrounded by hope and positivity.
- I am grateful for the support of my healthcare team.
- I am surrounded by positive energy and love.
- I am filled with strength and resilience.
- I am grateful for the kindness of strangers.
- I am surrounded by hope and possibility.
- I am grateful for the moments of joy.
- I am surrounded by people who uplift me.
- I am filled with hope for the future.
- I am grateful for the love of my pets.
- I am surrounded by positivity and encouragement.
- I am filled with gratitude for the present moment.
- I have the power to fight this with all I've got.
- I believe in the healing power of my body.
- I am grateful for each day of life.
- I am strong enough to overcome any obstacle.
- I have the power to choose my thoughts and feelings.
- I believe in the strength and resilience of my spirit.
- I am grateful for the love and support of my family.
- I am capable of finding joy and happiness every day.
- I have the power to stay positive in difficult times.
- I believe in the importance of self-care and self-love.
- I am grateful for the beauty of nature and the world.

Day 3 - Morning Affirmations

Say the following affirmations out loud, two or three times with increasing conviction and belief.

- I am confident in my ability to heal and recover.
- I have the power to visualize my way to health.
- I believe in the importance of laughter and humor.
- I am grateful for the opportunity to grow and learn.
- My higher power is working miracles in my life.
- I trust that the universe is bringing me what I need.
- I am strong, resilient, and capable of overcoming any challenge.
- I have faith in the power of love and positivity to heal.
- I trust that I am on the right path towards healing.
- I am surrounded by the love and support of those around me.
- I have faith in the resilience and strength of my body.
- I trust that I am capable of achieving my healing goals.
- I am courageous and brave in the face of adversity.
- I have the power to set and achieve my goals.
- I believe in the power of positive affirmations and self-talk.
- I am grateful for the simple pleasures in life.
- I am resilient and can bounce back from setbacks.
- I have the power to choose my attitude and outlook.
- I believe in the power of prayer and positive energy.
- My higher power is sending me love and healing energy.
- I am grateful for the kindness and compassion of others.
- I am filled with love and gratitude for my body.
- I have the power to cultivate inner peace and calm.
- I believe in the power of visualization and meditation.
- I am grateful for the moments of beauty and grace.
- I am strong and powerful, even in the face of illness.
- I have the power to inspire others with my journey.
- I believe in the importance of forgiveness and letting go.
- I am grateful for the moments of connection with others.
- I am surrounded by love and positive energy.

Day 3 - Evening Affirmations

Say the following affirmations out loud, two or three times with increasing conviction and belief.

- A higher power is surrounding me with love and light.
- My body is becoming healthier and stronger every day.
- Every cell in my body is filled with healing energy.
- I am capable of finding beauty and goodness in the world.
- A higher power is filling me with hope and positivity.
- My body is healing, and I am becoming more vibrant every day.
- Every cell in my body is responding to positivity and love.
- I am strong, brave, and unstoppable in the face of adversity.
- A higher power is helping me to find strength and courage.
- My body is a temple of health, and I am treating it with care.
- Every cell in my body is working to restore balance and harmony.
- I have the power to find meaning and purpose in life.
- I believe in the importance of rest and self-care.
- I am grateful for the power of hope and optimism.
- I am capable of finding joy and happiness in each day.
- I have the power to let go of fear and anxiety.
- I believe in the power of community and support.
- I am grateful for the moments of peace and serenity.
- I am filled with strength and resilience to face any challenge.
- I have the power to live each day to the fullest.
- I believe in the importance of self-compassion and self-forgiveness.
- I am grateful for the power of love and connection.
- I am confident in my ability to overcome any obstacle.
- I have the power to create a positive and fulfilling life.
- I can feel the support and love of those around me.
- The universe is guiding me towards health and vitality.
- Every day, I am becoming more resilient and determined.
- I am strong, brave, and capable of achieving my goals.
- I can feel the power of positive affirmations working within me.
- The universe is filled with infinite possibilities for my healing.

Day 4 - Morning Affirmations

Say the following affirmations out loud, two or three times with increasing conviction and belief.

- Every day, I am surrounded by love and positivity.
- I believe in the power of positive thinking and affirmations.
- I am grateful for the gift of life and all its blessings.
- I am strong and capable, even in the face of adversity.
- I have the power to see beauty and goodness in the world.
- I believe in the importance of gratitude and appreciation.
- I know I am capable of facing this challenge.
- I feel the love and support of those around me.
- I am grateful for the opportunity to grow and learn.
- I am strong, brave, and capable of overcoming anything.
- I know I have the power to heal my body.
- I feel the healing energy of the universe within me.
- I am grateful for the beauty and goodness in life.
- I am filled with gratitude for the blessings in my life.
- I know I am surrounded by positive energy and light.
- I feel the support and encouragement of my loved ones.
- I am grateful for the opportunity to experience life fully.
- I am strong, courageous, and unstoppable.
- I know I can find joy and happiness in any circumstance.
- I feel the strength and power of my inner self.
- I am grateful for the moments of peace and calm.
- I am filled with gratitude for the blessings in my life.
- I am worthy of abundance, joy, and peace.
- I am strong, resilient, and capable of overcoming anything.
- My entire being is filled with the power of positivity.
- I am surrounded by the love and support of those around me.
- I am worthy of love, acceptance, and forgiveness.
- I am filled with the hope and optimism of a brighter future.
- My entire being is becoming more vibrant and alive every day.
- I am surrounded by the beauty and wonder of the natural world.

Day 4 - Evening Affirmations

Say the following affirmations out loud, two or three times with increasing conviction and belief.

- I am filled with gratitude for the love of my pets.
- I know I have the power to heal my mind and body.
- I feel the love and support of the universe surrounding me.
- I am grateful for the beauty and wonder of the world.
- I know I am a warrior, strong and resilient.
- I feel the peace and calm of my inner self.
- I am grateful for the kindness and compassion of others.
- I am confident in my ability to fight and win this battle.
- I know I have the power to create a positive future.
- I feel the hope and optimism that comes from within.
- I am grateful for the simple pleasures in life.
- I am strong, resilient, and capable of overcoming adversity.
- I know I am surrounded by love and positive energy.
- I feel the hope and positivity that comes from within.
- I know I have the power to create a life filled with love and joy.
- I feel the strength and power of my inner spirit.
- I am grateful for the moments of beauty and grace.
- I am strong, courageous, and determined to win this battle.
- I know I can find peace and happiness in any situation.
- I feel the healing energy of the universe flowing through me.
- I am grateful for the love and support of my friends.
- I am filled with gratitude for the moments of laughter and joy.
- I know I have the power to create a fulfilling and purposeful life.
- I feel the peace and serenity of my inner being.
- I am grateful for the love and kindness of strangers.
- I am strong, brave, and capable of facing any challenge.
- I know I am surrounded by positivity and light.
- I feel the hope and positivity that comes from within.
- I am grateful for the moments of connection and understanding.
- I am filled with gratitude for the moments of peace and calm.

Day 5 - Morning Affirmations

Say the following affirmations out loud, two or three times with increasing conviction and belief.

- I know I have the power to live each day with love and joy.
- I feel the strength and resilience of my inner self.
- I am healing, getting stronger with each passing day.
- My body is resilient and capable of healing itself.
- I am grateful for the love and support of my caregivers.
- I am strong, brave, and capable of overcoming anything.
- I am healing and restoring my body to full health.
- My body is strong, healthy, and full of vitality.
- I am grateful for the moments of peace and calm.
- I am filled with gratitude for the love of my family.
- I am healing and restoring balance to my body and mind.
- My body is working hard to heal and recover.
- I am grateful for the kindness and compassion of others.
- I am strong, courageous, and determined to win this battle.
- I am healing and restoring my body to optimal health.
- My body is a miraculous machine, capable of healing itself.
- I am grateful for the support and encouragement of my community.
- I am healing and embracing a life filled with joy and purpose.
- My body is healing, and I am treating it with love and care.
- I am healing, my body is getting stronger every day.
- My body is a powerful and resilient machine.
- I am grateful for the love and support of my family.
- I am strong, brave, and capable of overcoming any challenge.
- I am healing, and my mind is becoming more peaceful.
- My body is healing and restoring balance to itself.
- I am grateful for the moments of joy and happiness.
- I am filled with gratitude for the love of my friends.
- I am healing, and my soul is becoming more vibrant.
- My body is fighting and winning this battle.
- I am grateful for the beauty and wonder of the world.

Day 5 - Evening Affirmations

Say the following affirmations out loud, two or three times with increasing conviction and belief.

- I am strong, brave, and determined to win this fight.
- I am healing, and my body is becoming healthier every day.
- My body is capable of healing itself with love and care.
- I am grateful for the kindness and compassion of others.
- I am filled with gratitude for the love of my pets.
- I am healing, and my spirit is becoming more resilient.
- My body is a temple of health and vitality.
- I am grateful for the moments of peace and calm.
- I am strong, brave, and unstoppable in the face of adversity.
- I am healing, and my mind is becoming more positive.
- My body is a miracle, capable of incredible things.
- I am grateful for the love and support of my community.
- I am filled with gratitude for the blessings in my life.
- I am healing, and my body is responding to treatment.
- My body is healing, and I am taking care of it with love.
- I am grateful for the opportunity to experience life fully.
- I am strong, brave, and capable of overcoming anything.
- I am healing, and my body is becoming stronger every day.
- My body is a powerful vessel of health and wellness.
- I am worthy of abundance, success, and prosperity.
- I am filled with the power of gratitude and appreciation.
- My entire being is responding to the power of positive visualization.
- I am surrounded by the love and support of my higher power.
- I am worthy of love, acceptance, and forgiveness.
- I am filled with the power of self-acceptance and self-love.
- My entire being is becoming more vibrant and alive every day.
- I am surrounded by the positive energy and light of the universe.
- I am grateful for the beauty and goodness in life.
- I am healing, and my soul is becoming more fulfilled.
- My body is healing and becoming more energized every day.

Day 6 - Morning Affirmations

Say the following affirmations out loud, two or three times with increasing conviction and belief.

- I am grateful for the moments of peace and serenity.
- I am strong, resilient, and capable of overcoming adversity.
- I am healing, and my body is becoming more vibrant.
- My body is a miracle, and I am grateful for it.
- I am grateful for the love and support of my friends.
- I am filled with gratitude for the moments of laughter and joy.
- I am healing, and my body is responding to love and care.
- My body is healing, and I am becoming more vibrant every day.
- I am grateful for the love and kindness of strangers.
- I am strong, brave, and confident in my ability to heal.
- I am healing, and my body is responding to positivity.
- My body is a temple of health, and I am treating it with care.
- I am healing, and my body is responding to gratitude.
- My body is healing, and I am becoming stronger every day.
- A higher power is guiding me on this journey.
- My body is strong, healthy, and capable of healing.
- Every cell in my body is working to heal and repair.
- I am filled with love, strength, and positive energy.
- A higher power is helping me to overcome this challenge.
- My body is healing, and I am treating it with care.
- Every cell in my body is filled with vitality and life.
- I am capable of finding joy and happiness every day.
- A higher power is supporting and guiding my healing journey.
- My body is resilient, and I am becoming stronger every day.
- Every cell in my body is responding to love and care.
- I am strong, brave, and capable of facing any challenge.
- A higher power is helping me to find peace and serenity.
- My body is powerful, and I am taking care of it with love.
- Every cell in my body is healing, and I am grateful.
- I am filled with positivity, love, and gratitude every day.

Day 6 - Evening Affirmations

Say the following affirmations out loud, two or three times with increasing conviction and belief.

- My body is responding to treatment, and I am grateful.
- Every cell in my body is responding to love, care, and positivity.
- I am filled with love, gratitude, and joy every day.
- A higher power is helping me to stay centered and grounded.
- My body is a temple of health and wellness, and I am grateful.
- Every cell in my body is working to restore balance and harmony.
- I am capable of finding peace and serenity in any circumstance.
- A higher power is helping me to embrace a mindset of gratitude.
- My body is healing, and I am becoming more vibrant and alive.
- Every cell in my body is filled with healing energy and light.
- I am strong, brave, and confident in my ability to heal.
- A higher power is filling me with love and positivity every day.
- My body is responding to the power of positive thoughts and energy.
- My DNA is programmed for health and vitality.
- Miracles happen every day, and I am open to them.
- Every cell in my body is working to heal and restore.
- I am filled with love, strength, and positivity.
- My DNA is powerful, and I am using it to heal.
- Miracles are possible, and I am manifesting them in my life.
- Every cell in my body is filled with healing energy and light.
- I am capable of finding joy and happiness in any circumstance.
- My DNA is responding to the power of positive thoughts and energy.
- Miracles are all around me, and I am grateful for them.
- Every cell in my body is becoming stronger and healthier.
- I am strong, brave, and capable of overcoming any challenge.
- My DNA is resilient, and I am becoming stronger every day.
- Miracles are happening within me, and I am grateful.
- Every cell in my body is working to restore balance and harmony.
- I am filled with positivity, love, and gratitude every day.
- My DNA is working to heal and restore balance to my body.

Day 7 - Morning Affirmations

Say the following affirmations out loud, two or three times with increasing conviction and belief.

- Miracles happen when I believe in them and work for them.
- Every cell in my body is responding to the power of positivity.
- I am capable of finding beauty and goodness in the world.
- My DNA is a powerful tool for healing and restoration.
- Miracles are happening all around me, and I am open to them.
- Every cell in my body is becoming more vibrant and alive.
- I am strong, brave, and unstoppable in the face of adversity.
- My DNA is a miracle, and I am grateful for it every day.
- Miracles are possible when I trust in a higher power.
- Every cell in my body is working to restore health and vitality.
- I am filled with gratitude for the love of my family.
- I am filled with love, peace, and positivity every day.
- My DNA is responding to the power of love and care.
- Miracles happen when I believe in myself and my ability to heal.
- Every cell in my body is filled with healing energy and light.
- I am capable of finding meaning and purpose in life.
- My DNA is a powerful force for good in my life.
- Miracles happen when I open my heart and mind to them.
- Every cell in my body is working to restore balance and harmony.
- I am strong, resilient, and capable of overcoming anything.
- My DNA is a miracle of nature, and I am grateful for it.
- Miracles happen when I let go of fear and embrace love.
- My DNA is a miracle of life, and I am grateful for it.
- Miracles happen when I stay positive and optimistic.
- I can feel the healing energy flowing through me.
- The universe is supporting me on my healing journey.
- Every day, I am becoming healthier and stronger.
- I am filled with love, positivity, and gratitude.
- I can feel the power of love and positivity within me.
- The universe is sending me positive energy and healing vibes.

Day 7 - Evening Affirmations

Say the following affirmations out loud, two or three times with increasing conviction and belief.

- Every day, I am taking steps towards better health.
- I am strong, brave, and capable of overcoming any obstacle.
- I can feel the healing power of nature surrounding me.
- The universe is conspiring to bring me health and wellness.
- Every day, I am filled with hope and positivity.
- I am capable of finding joy and happiness in every moment.
- I am capable of finding beauty and goodness in the world.
- I can feel the strength and power of my body within me.
- The universe is conspiring to bring me healing and restoration.
- Every day, I am becoming more in tune with my body's needs.
- I am strong, brave, and confident in my ability to heal.
- I can feel the power of my thoughts and intentions working for me.
- The universe is supporting me with the power of love and light.
- Every day, I am taking action towards my healing goals.
- I am capable of finding peace and serenity in any circumstance.
- I can feel the positive energy of those around me supporting me.
- The universe is sending me signs and signals of hope and positivity.
- Every day, I am filled with gratitude for the blessings in my life.
- I am strong, resilient, and capable of overcoming anything.
- I can feel the power of self-care and self-love within me.
- The universe is opening doors for me to find the right healing path.
- Every day, I am becoming more in tune with my body's signals.
- I am capable of finding meaning and purpose in my healing journey.
- I can feel the power of my breath and mindfulness in my healing.
- The universe is helping me to let go of fear and embrace love.
- Every day, I am surrounded by the beauty and wonder of the world.
- I am strong, brave, and capable of making positive changes in my life.
- I trust that everything is happening for my highest good.
- I am surrounded by love, strength, and positivity.
- I have faith in the power of positive thinking and energy.

Conclusion

Congratulations on completing a full week of positive affirmations! We hope that the daily 5-minute morning and evening sessions have helped you in your healing journey. By consistently practicing positive affirmations, you have taken a powerful step towards enhancing your mental, emotional, and physical well-being.

We encourage you to continue using this book by starting again from the beginning each week for as long as you need. Consistency is key to achieving the best results, and by incorporating positive affirmations into your daily routine, you can continue to tap into the power of positivity to support your healing journey.

Remember that positive affirmations are a complementary tool to medical treatment prescribed by your healthcare provider. By working together with your healthcare team and consistently practicing positive affirmations, you can take an active role in your healing journey and enhance the effectiveness of your treatment.

We wish you all the best in your healing journey, and we hope that this book will continue to serve as a source of inspiration, motivation, and positivity.

Made in the USA
Coppell, TX
26 July 2024

35191724R00015